CW00632007

Enlarged Tonsils Cured
by Medicines

BY

J. COMPTON BURNETT, M.D.

AUTHOR OF "DELICATE, BACKWARD, PUNY, AND STUNTED CHILDREN"

B. JAIN PUBLISHERS (P) Ltd.
NEW DELHI—110055

Price : Rs. 15 .00

Reprint Edition : 1999 2001
© Copyright with the Publisher
Published by :
B. Jain Publishers Pvt. Ltd.
1921, Street No. 10, Chuna Mandi
Paharganj, New Delhi - 110 055 (INDIA)

Delhi - 110 092

ISBN 81-7021-475-0
BOOK CODE B-2109

PREFACE

To those of us who have children
it is of some interest to know
whether enlarged tonsils should
be cut off, or treated by medicines.
Most medical men have made up
their minds that enlarged tonsils
can *not* be cured by medicines,
but must be cut off, and therefore for most people, professional
and lay, there exists no question
of enlarged tonsils, and whether
they should or should not be
removed.   But as for the past

twenty years I have treated my cases of enlarged tonsils by medicines, and have, moreover, succeeded in curing the great bulk of them, I am proceeding in the following pages to set forth my views on what to me is a very great question. If my views are correct, they will no doubt in the end prevail.

J. Compton Burnett, M.D.

86 Wimpole Street,
   Cavendish Square,
      London, W., *Midsummer* 1900.

Enlarged Tonsils Cured by Medicines

——◆——

IT is to some of us often a question of great interest and importance to determine, whether tonsils that have become enlarged should or should not be removed by operation. To start with, we may say that there are manifest advantages in operations for the removal of tonsils. It is soon over, and any benefit accruing

therefrom is at once enjoyed by
the sufferer ; he can breathe better,
more easily, and frequently soon
takes on a healthier hue ; and if
his pigeon-breastedness is only of
recent date, and costal ossification is
not far enough advanced to amount
to fixation of the ribs, the chest
rounds out and great improvement in patient's general condition
is presently manifest. Again,
swallowing is more easy, and all
concerned feel happier in their
minds when they reflect that in
case of inflammations and swellings
in the throat the chances of chok-
ing are much lessened. Moreover,
there is a good deal of satisfaction
in the feeling that the thing is over,
the job is finished, and one can

heave a sigh of relief, " Now that's done with!"

But is it?

I fear not.

And before leaving the question of the advantages of a mechanical removal of the tonsils, I would also name the diminution of the aggregate quantity of mucoid tissue thereby effected, and which is sometimes seemingly advantageous, much as we observe that the removal of a portion of the thyroid will improve the general condition of the goitrous. But as a minus of either is manifestly, at least, as bad as a plus, it does not seem easy to determine how much to excise. Still, granted that this happy middleway can be struck, there is conceivably advantage to be derived from lopping off some tonsil tissue.

I take it, therefore, that the advantages to be derived from the operative treatment of enlarged tonsils are as just stated.

On the other hand, there are certain unquestionable objections to an operative removal of the tonsils : there is the bleeding that occurs, at times with occasional danger to life, and the shock to the system and nerves.

Moreover, the administration of anæsthetics to delicate children is to be avoided, if any way possible. I have observed ill after-effects therefrom over and over again. Then there is the question of the functions of the tonsils, one of which I believe is to subserve constitutional asepsis. The ever-ready way in which the tonsils show symptoms of sympathy with constitutional ailings leads me to infer that they are often of vast importance to the integrity of the organism. The tonsils are nature's top-end outpost of the digestive tube, and as such are constantly at work to do outpost duty for the same. It is often stated that the tonsils, especially if enlarged, are a source of danger,* as affording an inlet to germs of disease; many disease germs certainly do impinge upon enlarged tonsils—

---

* "A very hotbed of infection" as was affirmed in my presence this very day.

that is manifest; and some have maintained that that is the very reason why said tonsils should be got rid of, inasmuch as said germs not only impinge upon the tonsils, but are said to actually penetrate into their parenchyma, there to thrive and multiply, and thence to poison the organism.

I am myself not aware that any real proofs have ever been given of the inward march of disease elements through the tonsils into the tissues. Many of the views held in regard to the mode of extension of diseases within the organism appear to me to be open to question. Thus it is the fashion to regard the various tubercular manifestations as extending from the periphery centripetally, but this I very much doubt. In fact, it seems to me that on the contrary the tonsils are charged with the function of defending the organism and protecting it. I lately was treating a case of syphilis, the primary lesion being on the right side of the glans. I tried to persuade the patient to leave the primary sore alone, so that it might be the last disease manifestation to disappear, for my experience teaches me that if the primary sore be maintained the inward march is much more mild, and less far-reaching — in fact, the constitutional disturbances are much more benign and of shorter duration. The idea that the primary lesion

is in itself the disease is false;
the real primary lesion is purely
mechanical, and the so-called
primary sore is really already a
peripheral expression of the constitutional poisoning. Have we
not had already the papule, the
vesicle, and the pustule, before
we get the Hunterian sore? How,
then, can the chancre be really
primary? The chancre is the
sore resulting from the burst pock,
which is now the peripheral expression of the poisoned organism, and,
if allowed to do so, the organism,
aided by remedies, quite overcomes
the syphilis-disease, and the LAST
expression of the disease is the
disappearance of the sclerosis a
the healing up of the sore th

originally came from the burst
pock.

I have repeatedly carried out
cures on these lines with the
highest possible satisfaction.

Well, the gentleman in question
at first consented to leave the so-
called primary sore alone; but a
neighbour of mine, a very high
authority on venereal diseases, was
horrified at my doctrine, and painted
to the imagination of our patient
fearful loss of tissue, and even de-
struction of the member; so patient,
as I commonly find in such cases,
insisted on the local sore being got
rid of, which I refused to do; but
I consented to watch and observe
the case; and very instructive the
purely observational *rôle* was. As

soon as the primary sore had been compelled to heal up, there appeared on the right tonsil a sore that could not be distinguished from the ordinary hard chancre, and proved very rebellious to treatment—in fact it is still going on.

But syphilis does not lend itself so well to demonstrate my point, though my own mind is quite made up in regard to its phenomena and cure. I have thought that chronic tubercular processes might be better adapted for my purpose, so before we enter any further into the questions that here concern us, we might with advantage inquire whether the mode of progress of certain tubercular processes is centrifugal or centripetal when we look at them in their clinical manifestations. In order to find out which way nature works I will take tuberculosis clinically, and by preference a few chronic cases, as more proof-affording than acute ones, for in chronic processes nature will generally be able to get her own way to a very large extent.

IN WHICH DIRECTION DOES NATURE WORK IN CHRONIC TUBERCULAR PROCESSES?

I wish at this place to determine whether we can find out how nature acts in chronic tubercular processes, viz., Whether we may regard the direction of the processes as from, or towards, the organismic centre?

It is needful to dwell a little, on the very threshold of this question, on the element of *time* in regard to *chronic* cases.

CHRONIC TUBERCULAR PROCESSES.

Chronic disease needs chronic treatment.

I lately read an account of a case of fatty degeneration of the heart having been cured in a few days. Last week a gentleman in good practice prescribed for a child with enlarged glands of the neck, and expressed the opinion that two or three weeks would see said glands completely cured. Incidentally my opinion was also sought, **and I** gave as my opinion that **between** two and three years **would be** required for their real **cure, or** perhaps even longer.

Remedies do not cure directly at all, but through the organic processes of nature. It is exceedingly difficult to fix the mind on the how and why of a given cure if of chronic nature, because after the medicinal stimulus has been given, we must bide a wee till nature mothers the action caused by the stimulus.

IS THE PHYSICIAN NATURE'S MASTER OR SERVANT?

Many have been the discussions in the history of medicine

as to whether the physician should be the minister or master of nature; it seems to me that *he should be both.*

It occurs to me that the physician is in much the *same position as a gardener*, who, for instance, wants to grow apples. Only nature can grow apples; but then it is crab apples that she grows unaidedly, not edible apples. No gardener can grow apples or crabs of himself, that has to be done by nature herself organically. But although no gardener can grow either crabs or apples of himself, yet, guided by human wit and experience, the gardener can compel nature to grow apples of the finest sorts and varieties;

he need not ask nature's permission at all, he merely arranges nature's forces so that she produces the apples required.

This, I take it, is the true position of the physician. It is only nature that can heal anything really, and yet nature cannot heal many things at all till the physician-gardener arranges her forces, so as to compel nature to grow apples in lieu of crabs; the physician's position is like an apple grower's further, in that nature requires *time* to grow apples; so also is it with nature's healing ways, nature requires time; and any attempt to cure in less time than she needs for her organic processes results in failure—absolute failure.

The element time in the cure of disease is not sufficiently considered either by medical men or by their patients.

These remarks are introductory to a short consideration of the treatment of chronic tubercular processes by *Bacillinum*, etc., so as to find out the direction of nature's way.

Whenever we have chronic ailments to cure, it is necessary to pause a wee bit and think, and we soon see that *the duration of the treatment must be proportionate to the time required by nature to effect her organic processes*, the sum of which makes up the cure.

It is commonly held that a tuberculously diseased part of an individual should be surgically got rid of, in order to prevent it from infecting the whole person, the idea being that the bacilli are the cause of the tuberculosis. The bacilli are the concomitants, and no doubt often the carriers of the virus which they very likely produce. Let us watch the behaviour of some chronic tubercular processes.

In October 1895 I received the following letter :—

"*10th October* 1895.

"DEAR SIR,—To-morrow, Friday, I intend to bring my brother to you for advice. He has had two operations—removal of leg twenty years ago in consequence of a white swelling at knee, and at Christmas 1894, removal of one testicle, in consequence of a swelling of a tuberculous nature. Since then it has attacked his other testicle, and another operation is advised; we seek your guidance in the matter,—Yours truly."

Patient's father died at sixty of tabes dorsalis, and his mother of apoplexy at forty-five. On examination, I found him in fairish condition, but very dusky; spits blood off and on for years; dulness under right clavicle; right leg amputated above knee; left testicle ablated, its position occupied by ill-healed scar; right testicle swelled, in its lower half solid, and on its outer surface three discharging fistular openings.

This gentleman's medical advisers were of opinion that though the case was hopeless by reason of the process having already gravely affected the right lung, still they thought the removal of the remaining testicle might prolong life, inasmuch as the testicle was evidently teeming with bacilli which had already spread to the right lung.

Let us consider this case, which has many points of importance. Now, if the infection had spread from the circumference towards the centre, the reasoning would seem to be sound, but is that here the mode of progress?

It appears to me that a bacillary invasion *may be* from without inwards, but in most cases I think the individual becomes qualitatively, potentially tuberculous, and nature, so to speak, picks up the bacillic elements somewhere within the organism where found, and bundles them off, away from the central organs and parts to, or towards, the periphery.

This point is of the highest practical importance as bearing on treatment, for if the process is centrifugal, surgical interference may be quite useless, and even harmful; and so in the case of enlarged tonsils, which is the point I am driving at.

I have thought the matter out, after carefully watching many clinical cases, and I find the trend of vital

processes to be from within out-
wards, and the peripheral manifestations are principally nature's ways
of turning the tubercular and other
elements out of the economy,
i.e., nature's midden-outlets from
the more important inside.

If any one will take the trouble
to watch nature's ways—say, in skin
diseases—he will see that even
where the first origin of the disease
is by infection at a given point
of the outside, the disease indeed
at first marches inwards ; but then
in the within great battles are
fought and many slain, whereupon
the organism reacts centrifugally
by carrying the dead and dejected
inside the camp to a point at the
periphery—*i.e.*, she ejects them.

I determined to act on this view, and began to regard and treat chronic cases dynamically from within.

This case—from October 1895 to the end of the year, all through 1896, all through 1897 and 1898 —was treated steadily and persistently with infrequent doses of *Bacil.* 30, C., *Tub. test.* 30, C., and some half-a-dozen other remedies, and at the moment at which I am writing, March 1900, patient is in good general health and spirits, and so he has been nearly all the time. At first his cough and blood-spitting lessened, and finally disappeared altogether ; neither lung has any trace of active disease now for very long, but the place, where the left testicle used to be, *opened and became fistulous*, in even pace with the healing up of the right lung and the disappearance of the cough, and this is still somewhat flickeringly active here and there, thus conclusively proving that the left testicle was the midden of the economy, which being ablated and forcibly healed up, nature then chose the right testicle and the right lung as her next least harmful offal pit. The surgeons who ablated the left testicle to save the organism have watched this case during all this time, urging for many months the terrible danger of delay in operating on the remaining testicle; and now that the patient has been well and sound of wind for very many months, they are of the same opinion still! Thus we see that a case of an admittedly tubercular nature, chronic, steadily progressing death-wards, was steadily left to itself surgically—dynamic doses of *Bacillinum* given at about eight-day intervals for several years, and the patient has slowly got well, and so remains ; the healing processes taking place in the inverse order of their appearance.

The tubercular process in the right lung was the last to appear and the first to disappear, then followed the right testicle, and finally the points of severance of the left testis.

I have watched this in a certain number of other chronic tubercular cases, and with the same result. So long as the peripheral opening is free to discharge, patient's life is safe, and if antibacillinic treatment be persevered in for many months, or several years, a genuine cure results. This is beautifully seen in fistula in ano, and in chronic tuberculosis of the tonsils.

Any close observer, if sufficiently patient, can convince himself that in the common chronic tubercular processes having a peripheral manifestation, the natural course which nature follows is centrifugal.

Thus, only two days ago, a young lady, niece of Lord X., was sent to me for treatment. Eight years ago she developed a strumous gland in the right side of the neck, an inch and a half below the ear; said gland was very neatly excised. Six years ago another lump was found at the same spot, this lump was also equally neatly excised, and now there is another lump come at the side of the very neat scar, also evidently a gland. That the thing is constitutional is thus clearly manifest, and this is made the more certain by the fact that menstruation now occurs every fortnight, and the glands in the right groin are found to be indurated.

It therefore follows that the treatment should be from within, and the local peripheral tubercular processes are to be regarded as outlets, and *not* as inlets, wherefore the ordinary surgical treatment of such tubercular processes is wrong and harmful.

CHRONIC COUGH. TUBERCULAR DISEASE OF LEFT ELBOW.

A single gentleman, thirty-two years of age, came under my observation on March 14, 1899, telling me that he had tubercular disease of his left elbow joint these twelve years. Six operations had been performed on the part, in Germany, during these twelve years, with the view of eradicating the disease, and thus saving the constitution, and with it the patient's life, but the seat of operation would never quite heal. Patient is well nourished, and I found his left elbow joint almost anchylosed, but an unhealing fistula exists at its side, from which mattery stuff is oozing. He is advised to have the whole joint excised, so as to be rid of the fistula. I advised, on the contrary, that internal treatment was the real thing to do. Patient consented, and placed himself frankly under my care for that purpose.

I began with a month of *Bacill.* C.

April 11.—Less discharge from the fistula.

Rep.

May 8.—I notice that the cough is worst in the morning, and in my experience the exclusively *morning* cough is often vaccinosic, and, moreover, I find patient was vaccinated as an infant, and again at twelve or thirteen for the second time.

Ergo, Thuja 30 for a month in infrequent doses.

June 21. — The opening of the fistula is much dryer and shows a tendency to close.

℞ Rep.

July 25.—The fistula has healed, but only with a scab.

℞ *Bacill.* C.

August 22.—Well, save a very little morning cough.

℞ *Thuja* 30.

October.—He is quite well, and with friends in Germany.

April 5, 1900.— Remains quite well ; no cough, and the elbow has quite healed, and he has increased in weight.

From this case it seems to me that the nature of the ailment was vaccinosis implanted on tuber-culosis, and that, moreover, the two existed side by side, each as a separate biosis, working from the centre towards and into the periphery.

CHRONIC STRUMOUS GONITIS.

A clergyman's son, thirteen years of age, was carried into my consulting room on June 12, 1899.

Rather pale, big for his age, well-grown, but his right knee had long been the seat of strumous disease. The knee three-fourths anchylosed, and at its side a sore place, whence came oozing matter from the diseased joint.

Leading surgeons, seeing no hope of a cure other than by operation, recommended resection, which was about to be performed. Patient had been troubled thus for a number of years, and all concerned were more than willing that an operation should put an end to the wretched thing.

At the end of four months, all the time under *Bacill.* 30, in infrequent doses, all discharge ceased, and in ten months from commencing the treatment, the knee was quite healed, and the lad in every respect in capital condition.

Movements are now being used to see if the amount of motion of the joint can be increased, which seems probable.

My point is, that the disease was of the constitution and from the centre to the outside, in which manner it was also cured.

Having now dwelt in a general manner on nature's ways in chronic disease, how she works from the within towards the outside, and that time is of the essence of these workings, I will now proceed to my task and give some examples of cases of enlarged tonsils cured by medicines ; they are not hearsay cases, but such as I have seen and cured myself.

ENLARGED TONSILS.

Cecil, æt. eight, was brought to me by his mother on May 20, 1897, for enormously enlarged tonsils, pains in stomach after food, snoring

at night, with restless sleep, dull
and stupid. He was nearly three
years under me, and then discharged
in excellent health. After one
month under *Thuja* 30, my note is
"vast improvement." The improvement continued under *Bacillinum.* "He sleeps quietly and
works better at school."

He came to me a few times in
1898 and in 1899, and when his
mother brought him to me for my
final inspection, I had the great
satisfaction of observing a fine
healthy lad, with tonsils long since
restored to their normal size and
functions. The boy has lost his
stupid look and takes a good position at his school.

ENLARGED TONSILS AND ENURESIS
CURED BY MEDICINES.

Whether the tonsils stand in any relationship of a peculiar nature with the root of the bladder or testicles has not been demonstrated.

Prosser James used to teach that the ovaries and the tonsils have vital connections, and we know of the behaviour of the parotid glands and the testicles in cases of mumps. The parotid glands and the tonsils are certainly pretty near physiological relations as well as neighbours anatomically.

A lad of sixteen was brought to me on January 12, 1897, suffering from "he wets his bed some-

times, and his tonsils are enormous,"
the right one being the larger. Many
of his lymphatic glands are indurated, and he also suffers somewhat
from eczema. He was discharged
cured at the end of 1899, though
his enuresis had long been well
before then, and also his tonsils, but
the eczema persisted till then, and
in fact there are traces of it still.

He had a number of remedies,
Luet. C. and *Thuja* 30 did perhaps
the most good.

Where a case is of deep-going
constitutional nature, it can only
be cured by a series of remedies ;
and when the thing is cured, it is
further of only historic interest.
It is very difficult to say exactly
how much of the curing was done

by each separate medicine; so here.

ENLARGED TONSILS AND ADENOID GROWTHS—SOMNAMBULISM.

Master X., ten years of age, was brought to me by his mother on October 19, 1899. He had been operated on for adenoids two years ago, but with no benefit. He has a chronic discharge from right ear, of which he is deaf; is stupid, cannot learn his lessons; sleeps very restlessly, and is often found walking in his sleep, causing much alarm and anxiety.

℞ *Thuja* 30.

Nov. 16.—He is better, and his schoolmaster reports him a little less stupid.

To continue with the *Thuja* 30.

Jan. 11, 1900. — His sleep-walking is very bad; the right ear runs very much; his violent outbursts less frequent.

℞ *Luet.* C.

Feb. 8. — The improvement in his powers of learning is reported by his schoolmaster to me personally as wonderful; no longer walks in his sleep.

℞ Rep.

March 17. — The improvement is increasingly manifest; tonsils nearly normal.

℞ Rep.

April 12.—The improved condition is more than maintained. I recommend his mother to keep him under my observation at certain intervals till the cure is consolidated.

I think it may fairly be conceded that the cure of an individual's enlarged tonsils by scientific medicinal treatment is incomparably better that merely ablating them.

Be it noted that not only the boy's tonsils were cured but the boy himself; he became mentally much more active and efficient, his sleep improved, his somnambulism was cured.

Be it also noted that a child with enlarged tonsils is in bad health otherwise ; the tonsils are not ill of themselves, but from the organism.

DEAFNESS FROM ENLARGED TO' S.

The deafness from enla

tonsils is often due not only to the obstruction of enlarged tonsils, but to the quality of the lining membrane of the Eustachian tubes, and adenoids in the naso-pharynx, so that the mechanical removal of the tonsils bodily, together with the adenoids, is often of no avail in these cases of deafness, nor does it suffice when the mucosa of the pharynx is hypertrophied.

Thus a boy of ten years of age was brought to me on September 1, 1889. He had been deaf for five years. His tonsils were removed by operation, but his deafness was in nowise improved. The boy was anæmic, readily took cold, and had had ophthalmia.

After *Morbill.* 30 there was

some improvement in his hearing, then followed *Scarl.* 30 for a few weeks, and on November 25 I wrote in my notes of the case—

" Hearing quite well ; he is altogether different ; his teeth are very soft."

℞ *Calcarea fluorica*, 3 trit., tales xxiv. One dry on the tongue at bedtime.

Long afterwards, on *Jan.* 22, 1898, he was reported as hearing quite well. It seems to me it is vain to expect to change the vital state of the tissues of the body by cutting bits off ; at most we can expect only such amelioration as may accrue from the removal of obstacles to normal processes. In the foregoing case the deafness was not due to the obstructing tonsils, and hence their removal had, as to the hearing, no good result. As the quality of the removed tonsils was certainly of the same nature as that of the linings of the pharynx and Eustachian tube, it must follow that most probably the remedies that cured the deafness would also have cured the tonsils of that which caused their enlargement.

ENLARGED TONSILS.

In the month of December 1896, a chubby little boy of seven years of age was brought to me for enlarged tonsils. His father had years before been a sufferer from fistula in ano, for which he was assured by eminent London surgeons and specialists there was absolutely no cure without operation, one going so far as to say that "any man who tells you he can cure fistula by medicines is a liar." I assured this gentleman that medicines given with much patience would most probably cure his fistula. He put himself under me, and I cured his fistula with medicines.

Now he is told the same story about his son's tonsils, which I entirely deny, and maintain that enlarged tonsils can be cured by medicines alone. This lad was under my care till the end of 1897, when his tonsils were, in his parents' opinion, quite well.

Patient was thus a year under

the influence of remedies. First he had *Tub. test.* C.; then a month under *Thuja* 30, then for two or three months under *Tub. test.* C., and finally *Bacillinum* 30 finished the cure.

I purpose going a little further into the uses of the large number of known homœopathic remedies for enlarged tonsils. There are a good many of them, and many thousands of cases of enlarged tonsils have been cured by homœopathic remedies; but the ignorant prejudice of mankind has pretty well laughed the thesis—that enlarged tonsils can be cured by medicines—out of life; so much so, that it is not thought quite the proper thing even in homœopathic ranks to admit that large tonsils can be lessened by gentle remedies. Just as I get to this point I happen to see the subject of the following case of

ENLARGED   TONSILS — ADENOID   GROWTHS—BACKWARD DEVELOPMENT.

A thin, puny boy, eleven-and-a half years of age, was brought to me on November 17, 1898, his father telling me that the patient was in a very unsatisfactory state; was thin, listless, apathetic, could not learn his lessons—his schoolmaster saying the boy was stupid and incapable of learning. His tonsils very large, bulging out under his jaw; naso-pharynx half filled with adenoids. No one could get an answer from him.

I have seen him every month, and now, after sixteen months' treatment, his tonsils and adenoids are much improved; patient has captured a good position in his school, is much praised by his master, and his father tells me how delighted he is to see the progress in every way.

I might go on and fill a big book with records of cases of enlarged tonsils cured by medicines, but for that I have neither time nor inclination.

When I first became convinced by practical experiment of the workability of the law of likes in the cure of disease, I took the trouble to read the history of the good work done by the veteran practitioners in old files of their journals, and I must confess that the present race of homœopathic practitioners compare very unfavourably with those of twenty, thirty, and forty years ago.

Many years ago *Baryta carb.* 30 or 12 was in very high repute for the cure of enlarged tonsils. Its reputation was well founded, as I can testify. Taken by itself, it is the biggest tonsil medicine we have. Where the tonsils have enlarged from vaccinosis, *Baryta* will not do much until the vaccinosic quality has been got rid of by *Thuja*, or *Silicea*, or what not.

Similarly, where the tuberculosic

quality lies behind, *Bacill.* is
needed first, and then the *Baryta*,
and so on.

The old practitioners cured enlarged tonsils with relative facility,
but then they followed a live
pathology of enormous value in
clinical life. They regarded the
tonsils as belonging to the living
individual who is ill; for his tonsils
are swelled — people that are well
do not get enlarged tonsils. But
in these clever days, when we
doctors know so much better than
the Great Architect what our
anatomical parts are good for, we
have decreed that the tonsils are of
no great service—in fact no good at
all—and, indeed, not only no good,
but actually in the way; moreover,

they are nasty little lumps that stick in our throats just for the purpose of catching disease germs and impeding our breathing, in fact, the tonsils are nothing but a nuisance, and the sooner they are lopped off and cast away the better. That being the creed of the great bulk of learned doctors, why should any one waste his time trying to mend medicinally such wretched odd bits as the tonsils. Why indeed?

Well, generally speaking, we don't! Just a few give a few doses of *Baryta* 1 for a few days, or may be weeks, and if the *Baryta* has not cleared them right away by our next visit, we are rather pleased than otherwise, for did we not always say that enlarged tonsils could not be cured by medicines, and that *Baryta* was no good in tonsillitis?

MY PRIVATE VIEW OF THE TONSILS.

There are views private and public, and my private view of the tonsils is as follows :—

They are placed on either side of the fauces for the primary purpose of lubricating the food as it passes along, and so prepare it for its passage down the gullet into the stomach proper. That the tonsils actually do lubricate the food can be tested by any one so disposed, unless he has lessened his organic integrity by having them removed, or unless disease has done it for him. A pair of good, healthy, well-formed tonsils is a rare sight indeed, it is quite pretty to see them when normal.

The tonsils lie at the top of the digestive tube, and whenever certain parts or portions of the body have to deal with something harmful, the same is passed along the circulation to the tonsils to be cast out, and the tonsils then act vicariously for said parts from elsewhere. A great advantage in having it cast out at the top of the gullet is that what is cast out at that part may be rolled up in the food and so rendered harmless, and if it is disposed to decay, it is disinfected by the gastric juice. In fact, an evil-disposed particle of anything sent by the economy to the tonsils to be dealt with, has

a very poor chance of doing any
harm in its journey from throat
to anus.

The various ~~hilings~~ of the
tonsils are for the most part not
on their own account, but for and
on behalf of the organism or one
of its parts.

During the past two years I
have watched several cases of
phthisis *cured* by the tonsils,—that
is to say, a series of abscesses
formed in the tonsils, each going
through the various stages of heat,
inflammation, swelling, suppuration,
and bursting, and had these de-
generative processes been in the
lungs or bowels, they would have
been of great and serious moment.
But being in the tonsils, they were

slowly sacrificed for the organism, and the patients' lives were saved, and also their health. The organism works from its centre towards the periphery and into the tonsils, which cast out. An uninjured tonsil is clothed with epithelial cells, and these form a perfect protection against infection from without. I have never seen any real proof that uninjured tonsils take up disease germs ; in fact, I do not believe it, and not only do I not believe the tonsils guilty of carrying in infection from without, but, on the contrary, they are specially arranged to defend themselves and the organism against outside enemies, and all the ailments and diseases that I have ever encountered in the tonsils have come from the within of the organism. The life and the diseases of the tonsils come from within, and they are but useful servants of the organism, and always at their post.

In curing tonsillary enlargements, it is often necessary to find out the causes of such enlargements. Thus in rheumatic tonsillitis the rheumatic state of the person should be mended, and therewith the tonsillitis. The statement that rheumatic fever has been known to follow tonsillitis—that is true enough. The inference usually drawn is, that had there been no tonsils there would have been no rheumatic fever. I read the pheno-mena the other way. Had the tonsils been stronger and more adequate, they would have borne the whole burden of the rheumatism, and there would have been no fever.   It is highly probable that minor degrees of rheumatism are arrested by the tonsils, and there dealt with, and that their function is very largely vicarious, protective of the organism and its parts.

DEAFNESS DUE TO ENLARGED TONSILS.

In the course of the year 1899, Miss E. T., æt. 13, was brought to me by her mother, telling me that patient was deaf from enlarged tonsils, and that her doctor had ordered their removal.   I could only find one enlarged lymphatic gland on the left side of the neck. This was her vaccination side, and the lassie being strong and otherwise in good health, I thought we had to do with a simple case of vaccinosic hypertrophy of the tonsils.

In a few weeks the tonsils went down and her hearing was quite restored.

The remedy: *Thuja* 30, in infrequent doses.

It is not to be forgotten that a competent (or, at anyrate, orthodox and qualified according to law) medical man had declared an operation absolutely necessary. No medicines would, he said, be of the least avail.

Still *Thuja* 30 cured the case.

ENLARGED TONSILS AND DEAFNESS.

On September 23, 1889, a strumous girl of eleven years of age was brought to me by her mother for enlarged tonsils and deafness arising supposedly therefrom. The tonsils met in the middle, so that the uvula was in part invisible.

Thuja 30, *Bacill.* C, and one or two other remedies were given, when—

January 17, 1890.—" I do not see much difference in her tonsils yet."

℞ *Vaccinin* C.

March 12.—" Tonsils about the same."

℞ Trit. 3^x *Baryta carb.*, gr. iv. One dry on the tongue night and morning.

April 19.—The tonsils are distinctly smaller.

℞ Rep.

May 30.—No further diminution in the size of the tonsils.

℞ *Silico-fluoride of Sodium*, 3ˣ trit., gr. vj. One dry on the tongue at bedtime.

July 16.—Tonsils are considerably smaller. The case was cured by the spring of 1890, and the remedies that achieved this result were the foregoing, and then two months of *Phytolaccin* 3ˣ, two months of the third trituration of the *Silico - fluoride of Sodium*, and finally a two months' course of the third decimal trituration of the *Phosphate of Lime*.

ENLARGED TONSILS AND ADENOIDS
REMOVED BY OPERATION.

In 1899 a gentleman brought his
nine-year-old son to me for what
his physicians term Imperfect Development of the Brain. This was
supposedly due to enlarged tonsils
and adenoid growths. The boy
did not speak till two or three
years of age—indeed he cannot
articulate properly even now. He
wets his bed, and has a piled-up
cranium; but the point I wish to
bring out is that the influence of
the removal of tonsils and adenoids
is not an unmixed blessing.

He breathes better since their
removal, but since then he is much
more nervous; he squints, and is

very odd in his ways; he gesticu-
lates and assumes odd attitudes,
looking idiotic, and yet he seems
to me to have ample brain power.
He is cryptorchic. He hits his
mother on the face and throws tea-
cups at his parents, and throws
people bits out of window.

These nervous symptoms have
come on so very much *worse* since
the removal of tonsils, etc.

There appears to be no doubt
that there was very great exacerba-
tion in all his nerve symptoms sub-
sequent to the operation, though
the breathing was distinctly improved. I may, perhaps, be per-
mitted here to refer to my little
work *On Delicate Children* for
further particulars on this subject.

ENLARGED TONSILS AND INSOMNIA.

There are certain cases of enlarged tonsils historically readily diagnosed that will mend rapidly, and by rapidly I mean in a few months. Thus a gentleman brought his little girl of eight years of age to me in the fall of last year. The tonsils were moderately enlarged and also many of the lymphatics, but the most distressing thing was the girl's sleep. Here the amelioration was very great—in fact she was practically cured in six months. There was a period of two months under *Luet.* C. to start with, then *Thuja* 30 for a month, and the former prescription then repeated, when patient was discharged cured.

ENLARGED TONSILS AFTER REMOVAL
OF ADENOID GROWTHS.

A very delicate backward child was brought by her mother to me at the beginning of 1899, suffering from enlarged tonsils. Although the adenoid growths from which she had suffered had been removed by operation, still her eminently silly expression had not improved. She did not breathe nicely, a little phlegm in her throat see-sawed backwards and forwards without seemingly ever being got rid of. Though ten years of age, her eye-teeth are still absent. After three months of *Bacill.* 30, her intelligence very greatly improved; she breathed better, and without the phlegmy nasal state.

She was then a few weeks under *Thuja* 30, and then again another *Bacillinum* 30. Whereupon her eye-teeth at last appeared, and that quite sound.

There afterwards followed the same remedies repeatedly, and also *Sabina* 30.

Now, after thirteen months' persistent treatment by medicines, her tonsils are about the right size, the breathing is good, and patient is somewhat nearing the normal; she articulates now, and answers a question promptly, and her parents and their friends are struck by the very great change that has come over her. It is to be borne in mind that where the tonsils are enlarged that is not, as a rule, the only abnormality, for very commonly the enlargement is only one of the ailings of the individual. The tonsils are glands, and where one gland is swelled there are often many, and after all is said and done you cannot cut away disease with the surgeon's knife.

ENLARGED TONSILS

In the medicinal treatment of enlarged tonsils there are two main lines of procedure, and the first is to cure the cause of the enlargement, which is commonly not only not attempted, but it is not even thought of. For it must be manifest that to get rid of the cause of the enlargement is the prime consideration. If this be done the enlargements usually disappear — this is the best way. When you cut off a tonsil you certainly get rid of it, so you do if you shrivel it with gland tissue-destroyers, but the perfect cure is where the enlargement disappears under the influence of dynamic remedies : here the normal tonsils remain to do the work allotted to them within nature's cycle.

That this is really so may be seen in cases where the tonsils are not bilaterally enlarged, but only on one side, and in such other cases where the tonsils are enlarged at the beginning of the cure, but where only one tonsil will yield to a given remedy. Thus Miss Marjorie X. was put under me on June 26, 1899 for her huge tonsils; they literally held the uvula tightly between them, and breathing was distressing, and swallowing miserable. After the patient had been two months under *Thuja* 30, and then a month under *Bacill.* C., I find the following note in my record of her case.

Nov. 20, 1899.— " The left tonsil is no longer enlarged, but the right one is very large."

So we have here a rather curious find : under *Thuja* and *Bacillinum* one tonsil becomes normal in size while the other is still enlarged.

If we want to be quite successful

in the treatment of enlarged tonsils
by medicines, we must look away
from the mere tonsils, and re-
member that although the tonsils
are the thing complained of, the
constitutional cause of their enlargement is the real disease, and
this it is that can *not* be removed
by operation. Those who see the
mere enlargement, and give
remedies for such enlargement
merely — those practitioners will
mostly fail to cure enlarged tonsils
by medicines, and will have much
to say of the advantages of their
mechanical removal.

It is not at all a bad plan to
begin the course of treatment with
Sulphur 30; after a while follow
with *Calcarea carb.* 30, and in the

third place give *Thuja occidentalis* 30. Each remedy should have a month or two to develop its action, to do its work.

As a rule before these have done all their work there is evidence of amelioration in the child's health, and the enlargement has somewhat lessened.

Calcarea phosphorica — say 3^x — two or three doses a day follows well; indeed I have often been almost startled at the sudden improvement that will set in under its use : the whole child brightens up, coughs disappear, the intelligence awakens, the ribs stiffen, and the surroundings are well aware that something is being done for the enlarged tonsils.

The third trituration of the *Iodide of Mercury* will often rapidly and radically change the aspect of the enlarged tonsils.

Calcarea iod. 3^x is often useful in the abjectly strumous.

In puny boys whose testicular development is very backward—in fact can scarcely be said to exist at all—*Aurum met.* 3 trit. is, with me, an old and well-tried remedy; it may often be noticed that, as the testicles take on life and increase in size, *the tonsils diminish* in bulk.

Where the tonsils are very hard and there is evidently much sclerosed connective tissue in them, the *Iodide of Barium* will help.

In stubborn cases, it will often be necessary to recur again and again

to the same remedies, notably
to such remedies as *Sulphur* 30,
Calc. carb. C., *Thuja* 30, *Sabina* 30,
Bacillinum 30 and C., before all
the bars to cure are organically removed.

Sometimes *Baryta carb.* 30 alone
will rapidly reduce enlarged tonsils,
but alone it does not often suffice.

Hepar sulphuris is a classic
remedy in enlarged tonsils, and in
some cases *Silicea* is the remedy.

RHEUMATIC TONSILS.

Guiacum, Phytolacca, Salix, and
such anti-rheumatics come into play
in the treatment of tonsils whose
enlargements are of a rheumatic
quality. There seems a disposi-
tion to regard the tonsils as the

entrance door of the rheumatism into the organism. I am satisfied that this is entirely erroneous, and that, on the contrary, the organism endeavours to eliminate rheumatism from the organism by way of the tonsils, and it seems to me probable that it is when the tonsillary outlet is insufficient that rheumatic fever may result. not from without into the tonsils towards the centre, but from the organism out into the tonsils, to be cast away by the defecatory work of the tonsils.

The more I watch the behaviour of the tonsils, the more I am convinced that they are charged with an excretory, a defecatory function, and that they excrete things out from the organism, casting them out both at the time of swallowing food and also as a kind of lubricating trickle; such excretions pass with or without the food, down the œsophagus like corn down a shute.

Moreover, I think the bulk of the private troubles of the tonsils, *i.e.* their diseases, are vicarious for the mucous lining of the body.

I am satisfied from my observations that the tonsils are capable of sacrificing themselves on the altar of the economy by ulceration, till nearly or quite all the tonsillary tissue is gone.

The extension of phthisis to the organism from the tonsils from the exterior is practically

a myth. I am quite prepared
to grant that, given a strong dis-
position to tubercular disease, a
wounded tonsil might admit the
phthisic virus, and the organism so
become infected, but only through
an actual lesion of continuity, just
as it might be the case on any
other portion of the mucous surface of the body. I have frequently
watched phthisis of the tonsils,
as I believe, save the organism
from death, by gathering and discharging—gathering and discharging over and over again—much the
same as one may observe the
organism operate in like manner
through suppurating cervical or
other glands. The cases I
in my mind appear at first a-

hyperæmia, and then there is a
seemingly encapsuled mass, the
containing membrane looking like
fascia on the surface of the tonsil ;
it will take first one side and then
another, and will repeat itself at
intervals over a period of several
years, and in the end terminate in
the good health of the individual.
Whether unaided nature would end
by curing the organism with the
aid of a series of tonsillary gatherings and dischargings I am unable
to say, because I have treated all
the cases I have observed with
remedies, notably with *Bacillinum*
in high dilution.

There is always some blood from
these tonsillary gatherings when
they burst, and they usually cause a

certain amount of alarm. I have known experienced lung specialists greatly puzzled by these cases.

In conclusion, I will state as my opinion, based upon clinical facts as I see them in my daily work, that enlarged tonsils can be more or less readily cured by medicines withal the task is often tedious; and moreover, that *the tonsils are important organs of the body, that have as one of their functions the preservation of the life and integrity of the individual.*

And if this be so, it must be manifest that tonsils should not be cauterised or otherwise damaged by local applications, and that their total removal is an act of ignorant folly.

Some have regarded the tonsils as filters barring the entrance of disease into the economy ; we will now shortly consider this question.

THE FILTER THEORY IN GLANDULAR FUNCTIONS.

In the *Non-Surgical Treatment of Diseases of the Glands and Bones ; with a Chapter on Scrofula** by John H. Clarke, M.D., there is a portion (p. 5) that I commandeer bodily for the purposes of this treatise. Commandeering seems to have a certain relationship to stealing, whereas exchange is no robbery, and hence I give to the learned author

---

* London, James Epps & Co., Limited, 1894.

of *Diseases of the Glands and Bones*, two chapters from any of my published scribings in exchange for the here commandeered one chapter, and although Dr Clarke will be the loser, I trust he will for old friendship's sake declare himself content.

Dr Clarke says (pp. 5-14) :—

ANATOMY AND PHYSIOLOGY OF THE GLANDS.

In ordinary language a "gland" means a gland of the lymphatic system. It is in this sense that I use the term in the present treatise. Anatomically speaking, all the organs of the body which secrete definite fluids, such as the liver. the kidneys, the salivary glands, the

sweat and sebaceous glands of the
skin, and also some organs which
have no known secretion, as the
pineal and thyroid bodies, are
glands. But when the word gland
is used absolutely, it is the lymphatic
glands which are understood to be
meant.

The lymphatic glands are little
bodies varying in size from a lentil
to an almond, and are very widely
distributed over the body. They
are like so many "locks" on the
system of lymph canals, which form
a network of vessels spread over
the whole of the soft tissues. The
office of these vessels is to take up
the used-up materials of the body,
pass them on to the lymphatic
glands, which so act on them as to

F

make them again fit to be poured into the current of the blood.

In the ordinary course of events the glands are very well able to discharge their functions, but at times extra pressure is put upon them. When one has a gathered finger, instead of the ordinary amount of waste products of the part, there is a great increase, and some of them are of a highly irritating character. In consequence of this we often find a red streak running up the arm from the injured finger to the armpit, and in the armpit one or more enlarged and painful glands. This means that the irritating matters are being dealt with by the glands. These may prove equal to the strain put on them, or they may inflame and suppurate themselves.

On dissection the lymphatic glands are found to consist of a capsule, and an internal portion composed of pouches communicating with each other, and richly supplied with blood-vessels and nerves. The pouches contain "a molecular fluid in which numerous nuclei and a few cells may be found in all stages of development"—(Bennett). There are lymphatic vessels leading into the glands and others leading away from the glands. The lymphatic vessels are provided with valves which only permit the fluid they contain to travel in one direction, away from the surface in the direction of the heart. Those vessels which enter a gland open into the lymph spaces of the outer portion of the gland ; those which leave it are connected with the internal portion.

The distribution of the glands is very extensive. The chief localities in which they are found are the neck, the armpits, and the groins externally, and internally under the lining membrane of the abdominal cavity (peritoneum), and in the folds of it, where it forms the band of attachment for the bowels (mesentery), and in the chest along the larger bronchial tubes, at the root of the lungs, and at the base of the heart.

It will easily be understood that the function of this system of glands

and vessels is of very great importance. The apparently solid tissues
of the body are in a constant state of
flux, of building-up and of decay,
and on the regular discharge of this
process of interchange (*Metabolism*
the scientific call it) the health of
the body depends. It is one function of the lymphatics to take up the
waste materials of the tissues and
re-organise them, so far as they are
capable of it, for the rebuilding of
the same or other tissues. If they
act too sluggishly the tissues become
thick and unhealthy, and a state of
obesity, either local or general, may
result; if they act too energetically
the opposite condition of wasting
will ensue.

But they have another function

of enormous importance in the economy. I have spoken of the familiar instance of glands inflaming in the armpit when there is inflammation of some part of the arm or hand. The lymphatics, therefore, not only deal with the waste of the body, they attack the products of diseased action, and, so far as they can, destroy the virus of disease.

I will not rest content with my own authority on this point. The *Lancet* of May 12, 1894, reports a discussion on a paper by Dr Walter Carr, entitled " The Starting-Points of Tubercular Disease in Children." In the report of the discussion which followed I find the following :—

" Dr Routh pointed out the value

of the lymphatic glands *as a means of arresting the disease*, in the same way that the poison of syphilis or of a dissection wound was arrested."

" Dr Carr, in reply, said . . . he believed that the glands were usually infected near the primary source of infection. *He had no doubt that the lymphatic glands did act as filters and arrested the disease.*"

Closely allied with the lymphatics are the tonsils, which are looked upon by many surgeons as useless incumbrances (from the patient's point of view), liable to become enlarged from the slightest provocation, and good for nothing except for providing the surgeon with the work of cutting them out.

But even in regard to the tonsils some authorities in the old school are waking up to the fact that they may have been put where they are for some useful purpose, and not solely for the surgeon's benefit. I quote the following from the *Homœopathic World* of April 1893 :—

THE TONSILS.

In the *Revue Homœopathique Belge* of December 1892, Dr Martiny adduces weighty reasons against excising or even cauterising the tonsils. He quotes from a work (*Etudes Générales et Pratiques sur la Phthisie*) by Dr Pidoux, which was accorded by the Faculty of Medicine the prize of 10,000 fr.

founded by Dr Lacaye, and in which facts were adduced to show that in phthisical patients the excision of the tonsils materially increased the predisposition to the disease. Says Pidoux :—

"I act in regard to the follicular angina of phthisis as with hypertrophied tonsils, which I never excise, no more than I do the uvula in phthisics or in those who appear to me threatened with becoming such ; as also with anal fistula, skin affections, pains, leucorrhœa, etc., etc."

And further on he says :—

"Now it is quite certain hypertrophy of the tonsils is one of the most benign and most natural expressions of non - degenerated

struma (*des strumes non dégénérées*).
It is often such with all the other
characters of simple and nascent
scrofula, in infants and strong
adolescents, well formed, of healthy
colour, with the aspect a little
humid and full of juices. It must
be feared, then, that the violent
suppression of this primitive affec-
tion may be followed, in a predis-
posed subject, with pulmonary
manifestations of catarrhal pus and
still more retrogressive ultimates."

Dr Martiny adds that the above
entirely agrees with his opinion.
For a long time he has advised
neither removal nor cauterisation of
the tonsils; for he has discovered,
on inquiring into the antecedents
of consumptive patients, that a

large number had formerly sub-
mitted to excision of the tonsils.
For many years he has not met
with a case of enlargement of
tonsils that did not improve so
much under treatment as to render
their removal unnecessary.

Dr Martiny maintains that
though nobody knows exactly what
part the tonsils play as glands in
the economy, this is no reason for
concluding that they are useless;
and that "to excise, to lacerate,
to cauterise deeply an organ which
exists normally in the human
species and in a large number of
animals," has always appeared to
him the reverse of prudent."

I am sure my readers will thank
me for enriching my pages with

the foregoing, and what specially concerns me is Dr Clarke's
filter theory as bearing on my own
theory here, that the organism in
dealing with disease works from the
centre towards the periphery. At
first sight the two notions seem to
contradict each other, but I sub-
mit that this is only apparently and
not really so, for while the one
function of the lymph vessels is to
bring home to the blood what is
fit, the other function is to arrest
what is *unfit*, and this it does by
swelling up the glands, whereupon
the organism (beginning at said
swelling) sets about extruding it
towards the periphery and out of
the economy. The organism sends
the whole blood mass, good and bad

alike, right out from the centre all over the body to the uttermost parts and particles; the lymph course will not return the bad, but blocks a gland therewith to prevent its return to the general circulation. Thus I apprehend it is with the tonsils, which are composed of coils; if a poison impinges on the tonsils and is taken up, it does not get very far in the coil till it is arrested and a block ensues — swelling then ensues, and the organism extrudes the poison by means of a gathering which then discharges its contents *outside :* for a gathered tonsil when it breaks and discharges does so outside and not inside, inasmuch as the inside of the gullet is outside of the economy. It is not always remembered that the *inside* of one's intestinal canal is in reality *outside* the *organism*.

We all know that in the case of a quinsy when the gathering bursts there is not only local but also constitutional relief, and though the abscess burst in the night, unknown to the patient, and all the nasty discharge finds its way down the œsophagus into the stomach, no harm is done; the stomach must necessarily be endowed with no small amount of disinfecting power, for the patients suffer no harm, and soon call for food. The more I study the tonsils, the more I know of the organismic manifestations in them, the more I am impressed with their importance as vicars-general in pathological matters for the economy, in proof of which I adduce the fact that shapely normal tonsils are very rarely to be found in the adult, the reason being that during the upgrowing they have been sacrificed on the altar of the economy for its saving.

Hence it is that the pathological quality or qualities of a person can so often be read off, so to speak, like in a book, from the appearances of or on the tonsils.

INDEX.

———◆———

Adenoid growths, cases of, 40, 48.

    „   „   removed by operation not an unmixed blessing, 62.

Anæsthetics to delicate children, administration of, 8.

Aurum met. in backward testicular development, 72.

Bacillary invasion may be from without inwards, 23.

Bacillinum in chronic tubercular processes, and enlarged tonsils, 21, 26, 28, 32, 33, 35, 37, 47, 51, 60, 65, 66, 69, 73, 77.

Baryta carb. in enlarged tonsils, 50, 51, 52, 60, 65, 73.

Calcarea carb. in enlarged tonsils, 70, 73.

    „   fluorica in deafness, 44.

    „   iod. in strumous cases, 7

    „   phosphorica in enlarg tonsils, 71.

G

Carr, Dr Walter, on tubercular disease in children, 86.

Chronic tubercular processes, how Nature acts in, 15.

Clarke, Dr John H., on non-surgical treatment of diseases of glands, 79.

Cough, chronic, case of, 32.

Deafness from enlarged tonsils, cases of, 43, 58.

Elbow joint, case of tubercular disease of, 31.

Enuresis cured by medicine, 38.

Filter theory in glandular functions, 79.

Glands, anatomy and physiology of, 80.

    ,,   Dr John H. Clarke on non-surgical treatment of diseases of, 79.

    ,,   of the neck, enlarged, 16.

Glandular functions, filter theory in, 79.

Gonitis, chronic strumous, case of, 34.

Guiacum in enlarged tonsils, 73.

Heart, fatty degeneration of, 16.

Hepar sulphuris in enlarged tonsils, 73.

Iodide of barium, 72.

    ,,   mercury 72.

Knee, case of white swelling of, and tubercular swelling of testicle, 22.

Lady, young, with strumous gland, case of, 29.
Luet., in enlarged tonsils, 39, 41, 64.

Morbill. in deafness, 43.

Phosphate of lime in enlarged tonsils, 61.
Physician, the, is he Nature's master or servant? 17.
Phytolacca in enlarged tonsils, 73.
Phytolaccin in enlarged tonsils, 61.
Pidoux, Dr, on diseased tonsils, 88.

Routh, Dr, on the lymphatic glands, 86.

Sabina in enlarged tonsils, 66, 73.
Salix in enlarged tonsils, 73.
Scarl. in deafness, 44.
Silicea in enlarged tonsils, 50, 73.
Silico-fluoride of sodium in enlarged tonsils, 61.
Somnambulism, case of, 40.
Sulphur in enlarged tonsils, 70, 73.
Syphilis, 12, 14.

Testicle, case of tubercular swelling of, 22.

Thuja in chronic cough, 33.

   „   in enlarged tonsils, 37, 39, 40, 41, 47, 50, 59, 60, 64, 66, 69, 71, 73.

Tonsils, author's private view of, 53.

   „   enlarged, after removal of adenoid growths, case of, 45.

   „   „   and insomnia, 64.

   „   „   cases of, 36, 38, 40, 45, 48, 58, 60, 62, 69.

   „   „   two main lines of procedure in treatment of, 67.

   „   Martiny, Dr, opposed to excising or cauterising, 88, 90, 91.

   „   objections to operative removal of, 8.

   „   Pidoux's, Dr, treatment of, 88.

   „   removed by operation not an unmixed blessing, 62.

Tub. test., 26, 47.

Tubercular disease in children, Dr Walter Carr on, 86.

Vaccinin in enlarged tonsils, 60.

PRINTED BY OLIVER AND BOYD, EDINBURGH.